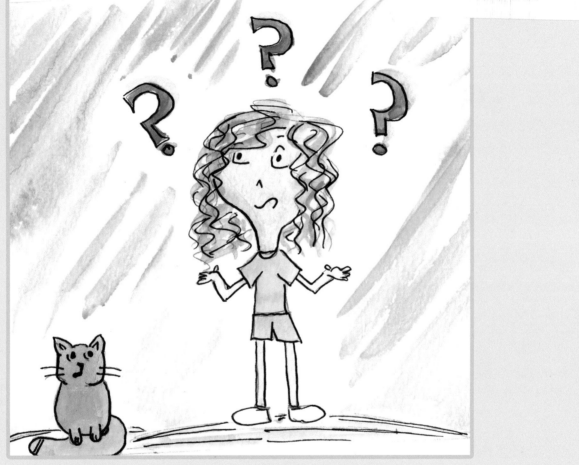

A G-tube you ask?
What is that, what can that be?
It's a gas-tros-to-my tube.
A fancy word for a fuel pump for me!

1

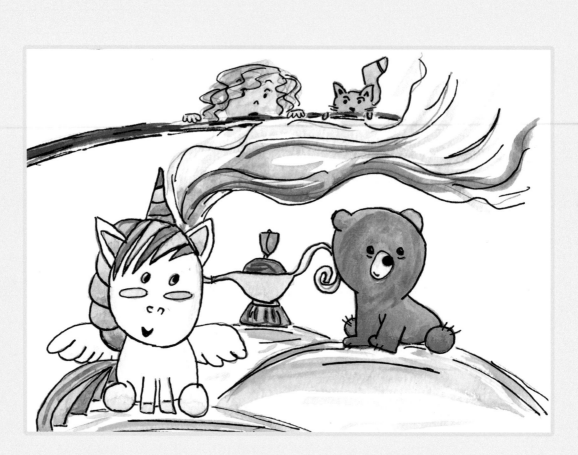

I think all of us children are special and rare.
Like rainbow unicorns, magic genies and purple polar bears.
We want to grow big and become fast, large and strong!
And we will, oh we will—
with a little help, we'll grow fast all along.

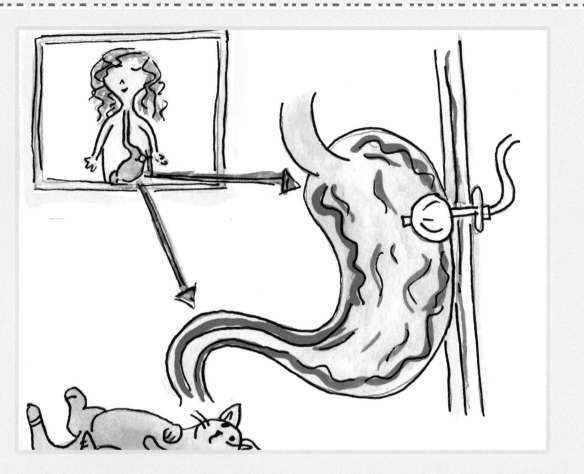

The first step is simple. You'll meet a doctor, quite friendly
Who gives you medicine to make you fall asleep,
so you'll sleep safely and soundly.
They'll put a tube in your belly,
while you dream of big airplanes or dolls.
And when you awake, a fuel pump will be attached
to your belly's wall!

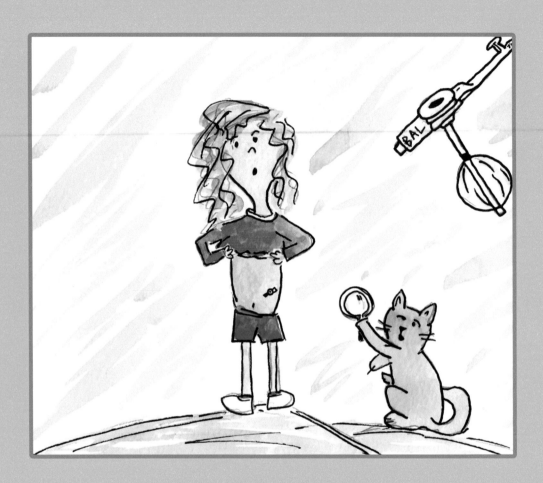

It will hurt at first;
feeling to me like a bug bite or new cat scratch.
But the more you move, twist and turn it,
you'll hardly notice your little fuel patch!
It'll sit on your belly like a cute button top.
Hidden under your shirt, invisible to even your Pop.

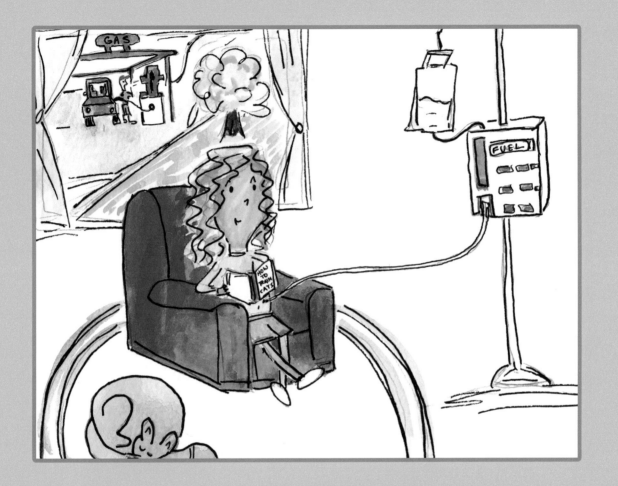

It's simply a tube like one a car needs for gas.
So, when we need food energy, we can fill us up fast!
We plug it in to our healthy formula to help make us strong.
And next thing you know, it gives us energy to be zooming along!

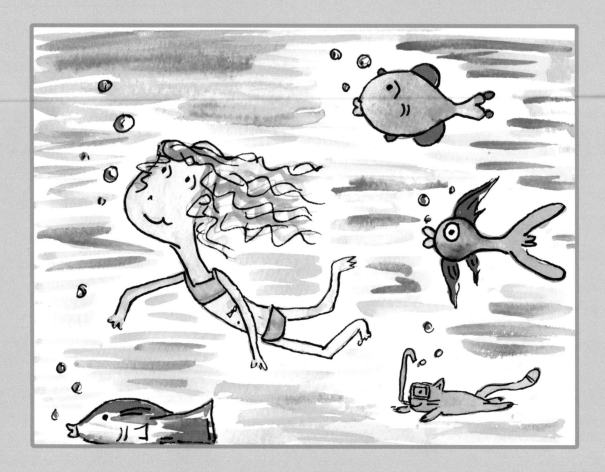

I at first was afraid and even a little bit sad.
But this fuel pump I tell you, didn't change me a tad.
It didn't hold me back, I still dance, laugh and swim.
Shoot hoops, bowl strikes and win races in gym.

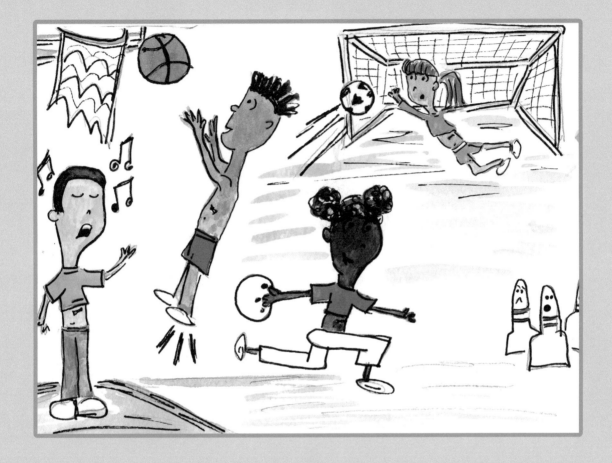

You may think you're alone but you're not. No you're not!
The amount of children with fuel pumps? So many! A lot!
Maybe you'll meet some of them soon, we shall see.
Until then remember this book and remember to think of me.

Now this has been fun,
and I'm sorry to go.

I have more kids to talk to,
to tell them what you now know!

That your G-tube will help you.
It won't slow you down.

Its job is to make you stronger
so you can zoom all around!

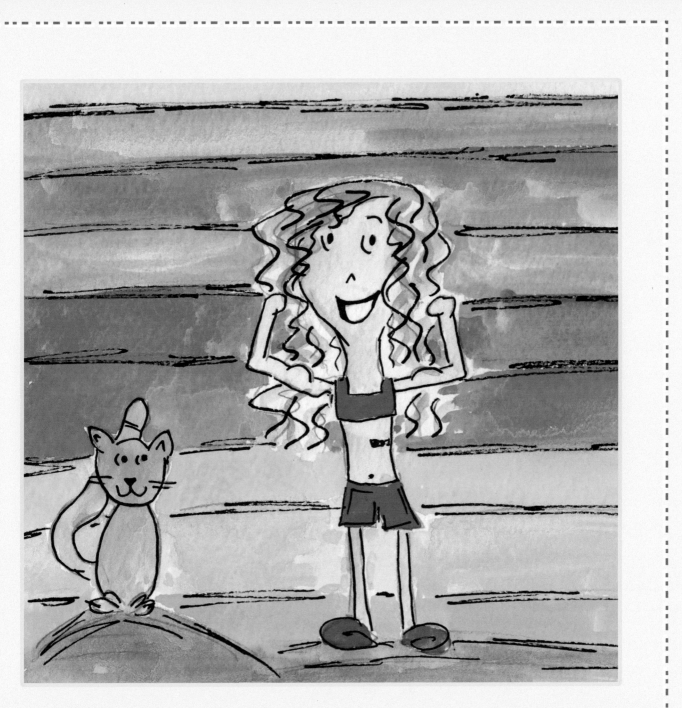

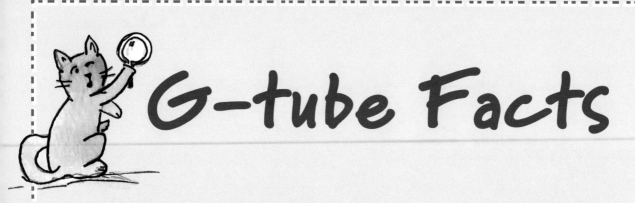

G-tube Facts

1. G-tubes are feeding tubes that are needed for many different health conditions.

2. The most common use is to help with **nutrition** when a child is unable to eat enough food by mouth.

3. G-tubes can also help **vent** the stomach for air or drainage when your child is bloated.

4. There are many different types of G-tubes. Some are '**buttons**' and some are longer tubes. All work in similar ways.

5. Some are put in surgically into the belly and held in place by a water-filled balloon. Some are put in endoscopically (using a camera)..

6. Over half a MILLION people in the United States have feeding tubes. Your child is not alone!

7. Kids can still do everything (even swimming!) that they did before the feeding tube. They may even have more energy and be more active!

Procedure Details

1. Your child will need to stop eating and drinking 8 hours before the procedure. This is called '**NPO**' time.

2. The procedure will take about 30 minutes to an hour.

3. The procedure can be done **laparoscopically** (with small incisions and a camera), **open** (with one larger incision), or **percutaneously** (small skin incision with '**endoscopy**'-a camera into the mouth).

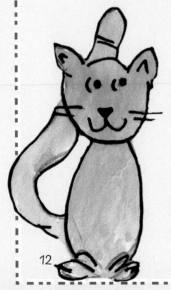

4. After the procedure, your child may stay in the hospital usually for a day or two.

5. Feedings can start the next day! A nurse will help teach you.

6. Your child may have stitches through the tube. These typically remain for 7 days.

7. Your child can bathe as usual the next day!

8. Your child can play normally too! Even tummy time is allowed!

9. All supplies you will need will be given to you before discharge or sent to your house. We will teach you how to do everything; do not panic!

10. Your doctor will see your child after 4-6 weeks and may change the G-tube at this time.

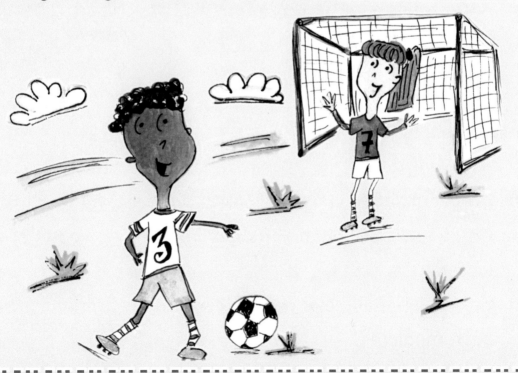

Basic Care

1. Always wash your hands before touching the G-tube!

2. Wash the site with soap and warm water daily. Keep it clean and dry.

3. Do not use scented lotions or ointments.

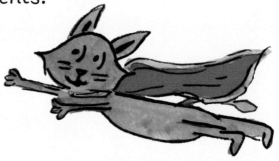

4. Flush with warm water (10 cc's)
   a. Before and after any feeding
   b. Before and after any medicines
   c. Every 8 hours

5. Medicines
   a. Ask your doctor what medicines can go into the G-tube.
   b. Don't forget to crush pills into powder and mix with water.
   c. Don't forget to open capsules and mix the powder with water.
   d. Give one medicine at a time and flush with water between each medicine.

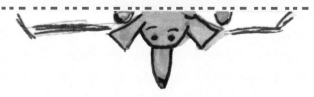

6. Clean extension sets daily with warm water. Allow to air dry.

7. Always know the size of your child's G-tube. It is written in big black letters on the top of the tube.

8. Check the G-tube measurement daily. Sometimes it can slip into the stomach too far and not work as well!

9. Check the balloon's water every week and refill as needed because water does evaporate!

   a. Usually the tube will become loose when the water is low.

   b. Refill with only distilled or city water.

   c. Do not use well water or saline.

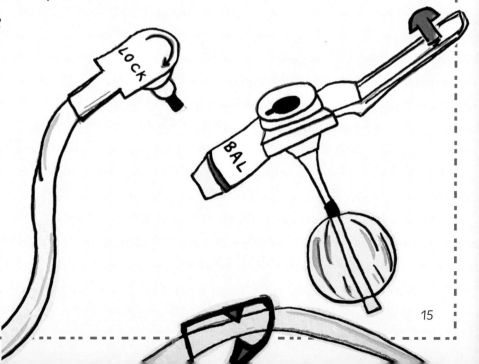

Feeding

1. Attach the extension tubing (if your child has a button).

2. Flush with 10-15 cc's warm water.

3. Attach the pump or syringe to the G-tube.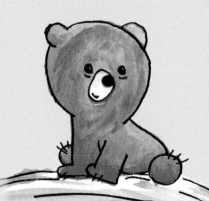

4. Unclamp the G-tube.

5. Start syringe or pump feed!

6. Flush with 10-15 cc's warm water again when finished.

7. Clamp the G-tube and close the little cap.

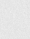

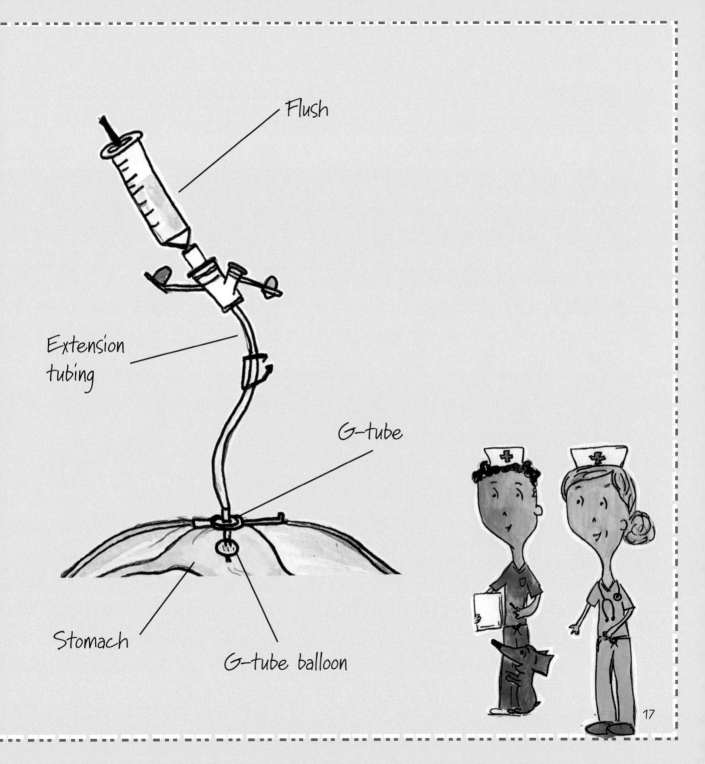

Flush

Extension tubing

G-tube

Stomach

G-tube balloon

Uh oh! What if...

Leaking, leaking, everywhere!

1. Don't worry. ALL G-tubes LEAK!
2. G-tubes will leak EVEN MORE if your child is sick.
3. You can use tape to stabilize the G-tube—this will help prevent leakage especially when it's healing.
4. Try placing gauze under the tube.
5. Sometimes a little blood leaks. This is normal too. If the bleeding does not stop, please call your doctor.

The tube fell out!

1. Don't panic! This is not an emergency.
2. If it falls out in the first 4-6 weeks (before your first follow-up appointment), go to the hospital immediately. Bring your G-tube supplies with you. Do not delay as the hole can close up within hours.
3. If it falls out after 4-6 weeks, you can replace it at home. Use a syringe to pull back on the feeding port to make sure you get stomach contents back. This verifies it is correctly in the stomach. If you do not see stomach juices, go to the emergency room.

We have a clogging problem!

1. Try flushing the G-tube with cranberry juice or Coke.
2. Put as much as you can into the tube and then clamp it for 2 hours.
3. Try flushing the tube again. If still clogged, call your doctor.
4. Never put anything rigid into the tube!

Granulation tissue? What is that?

1. Granulation tissue is extra dark pink or red tissue that forms around the G-tube.
2. Some people describe it as beefy or raw looking!
3. It is the body's normal response to a foreign object.
4. It can cause irritation and leakage.
5. It is very common! And not dangerous!
6. We can treat granulation tissue with special medicines so call your doctor.

I think it's infected.

1. The skin around the G-tube can get infected and be pink, moist, warm, and tender.
2. Try over-the-counter antibacterial or fungal creams. If there is no improvement in two days, call your doctor.
3. If your child has a fever, call your doctor.

Doctor Words

Gastrostomy tube (Your G-tube!): A tube that we place into the belly so that we can directly access the stomach for feeding, hydration, or medicine. When kids have trouble eating, this helps them get all the food they need.

NPO: Nothing to eat or drink starting at midnight the night before surgery because if you eat, putting you to sleep can be dangerous.

Laparoscopy: A type of surgery using small skin incisions to enter the abdomen and a camera projected on a video monitor.

Endoscope: A camera that goes into your mouth and travels to your stomach so we can see inside!

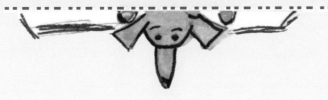

Hollister dressing: A large circular dressing that helps keep a long G-tube in place with a ziplock-type fastener.

Silver nitrate sticks: Special medicine that helps to remove granulation tissue. The silver burns the granulation tissue, making it fall off.

MIC-Key: A type of G-tube that we often call a 'button'.

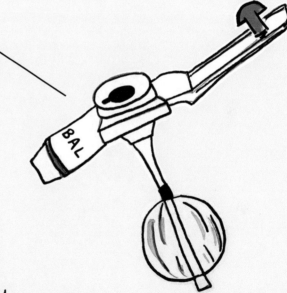

PEG tube: Another type of G-tube that is placed using an endoscope.

French Scale: Used to measure the width of each G-tube so they fit each child. Example: 16Fr.

Notes

Notes

Meet the Author:

Dr. Maria Baimas-George

Maria Baimas-George MD MPH is a surgeon, training to specialize in abdominal transplantation. Inspired by her patients and mentors, she writes and illustrates books explaining medical and surgical conditions to children and their loved ones. Her goal is to create books that provide useful information to help with understanding and to offer comfort and hope.

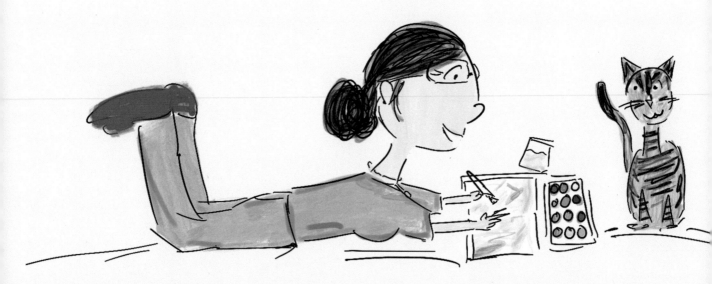